Deploying Dopamine

The Gateway Chemical
to a Happier & More Motivated Life

Christian J. Kalekas
Daliah H. Wachs

Illustrated by Kaytlin L. Kalekas

About the Authors

Christian Kalekas is receiving his education at Dominican University, majoring in Neurobiology with a focus on Neuroscience

Daliah Wachs MD, FAAFP is a board-certified family medicine physician and syndicated radio personality

**"Without dopamine,
desire died.
And without desire, action
stopped."**

James Clear, *Atomic Habits*

Table of Contents

Introduction

From ordering best-selling self-help books to delving into the latest dietary trends, the world seems obsessed with finding new ways to live a more fulfilling life.

The art of thriving as a human should not be confined to excelling solely in a singular aspect of life. Contemporary society would have one believe that meaningful success is waiting behind the next milestone or advancing to the next pay grade - but these are wholly insufficient and borderline destructive.

Although the idea of improvement can be vague and quantifies many aspects of life, the pursuit of these personal and societal gains is an inherent human inclination.

The concept of strengthening our weaknesses and finding the motivation to do so is crucial to living up to the high standards to which we, at times, set ourselves.

However, the one thing many of these "self-improvement" campaigns get wrong is the idolization of making only a singular change.

"Get rich quick with this one investment"
"Try this miracle pill and achieve your weight loss goal"
"Follow your dreams with our 5-step program"

These self-help experts continually sell the idea that making this one change will dramatically improve your everyday life.

Yet, this narrative only paints part of the picture.

Becoming the person you imagine yourself to be requires a collective amount of changes - not merely a singular one.

Making even one substantial modification to our lives can prove daunting, let alone the prospect of multiple changes.

How can we motivate ourselves to make these alterations to our character? How can we stack these seemingly inconsequential acts to build us into the character we seek?

Amid the preaching of self-help literature, motivational speakers, and life mentors, a single unifying element takes center stage: Dopamine.

How you feel right now, how you will feel an hour from now, and how you will feel next week is crucially reliant on our dopamine.

Our daily motivation and willingness to push through challenges depends on the intricate chemical process dopamine provides.

In this book, we teach you what dopamine is, when it dysfunctions, and the art of deploying it effectively when the need arises.

Chapter 1
Dopamine

To combat the increasing rates of obesity found around the world, the anti-obesity drug rimonabant was released to the public in 2006. Early clinical trials of Rimonabant showed significant weight loss and healthier waist dimensions unseen in the medical world to this point. Although rimonabant was rejected in the United States, 38 countries, including Brazil, Mexico, and the European Union, approved the distribution of the drug.

Marketed as an endocannabinoid antagonist, rimonabant was a drug that suppressed appetite and proved to be an effective method to decrease the chances for individuals to develop cardiovascular diseases. This so-called "miracle drug," as many rimonabant users claimed it to be, generated considerable optimism for many in the field as an effective pharmaceutical remedy for obesity.

Yet, just two years later, rimonabant was withdrawn and banned from public use.

How can a drug with as much excitement as rimonabant be completely off the market just a few years later?

While the drug exhibited promising results in the aspect of weight loss, rimonabant was also shown to inhibit increases in dopamine neural activity.[1] Many who had taken the drug saw adverse side effects that included depression, anxiety, and suicidal ideation. In a trial study, these adverse effects were observed at a rate twice as high among rimonabant users when compared to those who received a placebo.

This prompts us to question the relationship between our mood and the dopamine levels in our body. Could the drug's ability to halt dopamine production cause these unexpected side effects? Amidst all the chemicals and mechanisms our body uses, how can this singular chemical influence so much of our daily life?

What is Dopamine?

Dopamine is a naturally occurring catecholamine that exists in all living animals.

Catecholamines are neurohormones made in the neuroendocrine chromaffin cells of the brain and adrenal glands and not only include dopamine but also norepinephrine (noradrenaline), and epinephrine (adrenaline).

These catecholamines, including dopamine, act as neurotransmitters and additionally, they may act as precursors to other molecules. They are also released during our fight or flight response and

---

[1] Oleson, Erik B., and Joseph F. Cheer. "A Brain on Cannabinoids: The Role of Dopamine Release in Reward Seeking." *National Library of Medicine*, 2012. https://www.ncbi.nlm.nih.gov/pmc/articles/ PMC3405830/. Accessed 27 July 2023.

during activities we find pleasurable, such as sex, sleep, and eating.

Some have referred to dopamine as the "feel-good hormone" as it is a part of the brain's reward system. But the neurotransmitter and hormone serotonin also deserves credit.

As dopamine plays a major role in reward and motivation, serotonin plays a major role in one's mood and happiness. These hormones may interact with each other to maintain a chemical balance within the body.

This multifaceted system exists as positive feedback for what the brain perceives as pleasurable behavior.

When we engage in activities that bring pleasure, such as eating, socializing, or achieving goals, the brain releases dopamine. This surge of dopamine not only signals the brain to take notice of these activities but also motivates us to repeat them.

Evolutionarily this system we believe was designed such that species would procreate if they were engaging in an act, i.e. sex, that caused pleasure.

Now getting technical, dopamine is known as a neuromodulator. Neuromodulators are released at the synapses or gaps of nerves to convey a message. The message conveyed occurs at a receptor. When the receptor is triggered, a cascade of chemicals or hormones may relay more messages or perform a function.

Hence dopamine directs multiple pathways, communications, and functions in a complex and intrinsic system that we've only begun to understand.

How Dopamine Works

While various outlets can trigger the release of dopamine, its impact on individuals is influenced by a multitude of factors. Elements such as the intensity of the dopamine response and the duration of the pleasure sensation can also be shaped by these influences.

It is crucial to recognize that not all individuals respond similarly to dopamine stimuli due to differences in their baseline dopamine level—a set amount of dopamine that is circulating in your body at all times. This baseline sets the tone for one's overall mood throughout the day.

The baseline dopamine level is subject to variation among individuals based on genetics, behavior patterns, recent life experiences, sleep routines, and dietary habits.

Upon exposure to potentially pleasurable experiences, our dopamine baseline experiences spikes, commonly referred to as phasic releases. Moreover, instances of exceedingly pleasurable encounters, which trigger substantial or frequent phasic releases, can perversely lead to a drop in the baseline dopamine level.

The intricate system of dopamine necessitates proper management. The pleasure of a particular experience isn't solely dependent on the height of its peak; rather, the height of the peak relative to the baseline level.

To maintain a healthy relationship with our dopamine and maintain a generally good mood throughout the day, we must ensure that our baseline does not rise too high or too low.

Frequent encounters with elevated dopamine levels or the layering of dopamine sources may diminish the gratification derived from such exposures, similar to the concept of tolerance.

Additionally, our perception of a specific dopamine-triggering experience is also influenced by our past encounters.

Comparable to the waning of our emotional response after witnessing a home run or goal, our subsequent attentiveness and enthusiasm for ensuing plays undergo an involuntary decline for a specific duration.

This phenomenon explains why engaging in a repeatedly enjoyed activity can elevate the threshold for pleasure, leading to a diminishing sense of gratification over time.

This means the satisfaction we derive is based upon two primary components: our intrinsic baseline dopamine level and the frequency and magnitude of prior phasic releases.

A prevalent misconception is that dopamine is solely responsible for the generation of positive emotions and satisfaction. In reality, dopamine reinforces these emotions through the efforts of neurotransmitters such as serotonin, oxytocin, and endorphins.

Thus, it's a system navigated by dopamine, —a complexity that we can delve into, understand, and harness.

Chapter 2
Why We Need Dopamine

The main purpose of our and every other species on Earth is to ensure our survival. This fundamental goal relies on our capacity to endure and procreate.

In order to reproduce, we must not merely survive, but thrive in our environment.

Much like our Stone Age ancestors, who navigated the landscape in pursuit of essentials such as water, food, physical activity, relationships, and shelter, these factors collectively shaped our overall well-being and, most importantly, our ability to reproduce.

But how does the human species persevere in its pursuit of existence and propagate while having to navigate the relentless challenges we encounter in this world?

This pursuit, when accompanied by plausible motivation, can aid us in overcoming any obstacles. This motivating force is none other than the product of dopamine.

Imagine living in a world with no reward system. You work 50 hours a week but are not paid a penny for your labor. You dedicate hours of studying for an impending quiz only to fail. You sweat through daily mile runs yet see no weight loss. Safe to say, that no one would endure working in such conditions.

Such a world is hardly one any of us would willingly embrace. This is a world absent of dopamine.

When you take away the reward system, you take away a foundation of motivation. We humans are intrinsically programmed to establish a motive for work. Whether we set goals or are confronted with tasks, we instinctively link them to the potential benefits they can yield.

In 2023, 52% of Americans said their top New Year's resolution was to exercise more[2]. It's unlikely that the majority within this statistic enjoy the act of working out; rather, their motivation is rooted in the benefits that exercise provides. We want to look better, feel better, and live a relatively healthy life - and we know that comes through a consistent exercise regimen.

We've all encountered instances when the attraction of the reward overshadows the necessary toil the task demands. Why do you think a mere 9% of people who create New Year's resolutions manage to see them through?[3] It's because we disregard the actual hard work and dedication a goal requires to come true. We need to not only avoid underestimating the toil a goal demands but also create that much-needed motivation within ourselves.

This is why dopamine is crucial for us. Dopamine injects life with the "want" that propels us forward.

[2] Buchholz, Katharina. "Chart: America's Top New Year's Resolutions for 2023." *Statista*, 23 December 2022, https://www.statista.com/chart/29019/most-common-new-y ears-resolutions-us/. Accessed 7 August 2023.

[3] Batts, Richard. "Why Most New Year's Resolutions Fail | Lead Read Today | Lead Read Today." *Fisher College of Business*, 2 February 2023, https://fisher.osu.edu/blogs/ leadreadtoday/why-most-new-years-resolutions-fail. Accessed 7 August 2023.

Just as we saw in rimonabant users, our emotions and the way we perceive ourselves and the world around us are heavily dependent on this chemical.

Dopamine appears everywhere in our lives, and the fundamentals of our dopamine system are desire, motivation, and reward.

Desire

Dopamine drives desire.

Desire can be as simple as craving a piece of chocolate late at night or as ambitious as aspiring to graduate at the top of your class.

Desire, when approached the correct way, can provide substantial benefits to one's life:

- The desire to improve your marriage

- The desire to help your community

- The desire to become the best player on the team

Desire, or the "wanting" of something, can be related to many thoughts in our daily lives. Often acting as the initial spark towards achieving a goal, we must acknowledge that our desires inevitably remain unfulfilled if not accompanied by action.

Motivation

Motivation is action.

What distinguishes us now from the person we aspire to be is the willingness to transform desires and ideas into action.

Motivation can be hard to come by, but those who create their own motivation typically find more success. This work or action is what makes our desires obtainable:

- The desire to improve your marriage
↓
You designate one day in the week for a "Date Night"

- The desire to help your community
↓
You volunteer on weekends to help with the local homeless shelter

- The desire to become the best player on the team
↓
You perform extra reps before and after practice

Reward

Reward creates ambition.

The reward system and the release of dopamine
are directly related.

Perhaps you've experienced a similar scenario:
someone hints at having a gift for you, and
immediately your thoughts wander towards the
exciting possibilities of what it could be. Once you
receive the gift, you eagerly unveil it, only to
discover an ordinary pen within. While this example
might seem somewhat exaggerated, we're all
familiar with that surge of anticipation cut off by
reality. This feeling of being let down is the result of
our dopamine levels crashing.

This works oppositely as well. When shocked by a
surprise birthday party or handed the keys to a new
car on our sixteenth birthday, our expectations were
surpassed, and dopamine levels spiked.

By attaching realistic rewards to a task, we are
more inclined to finish that task.

- The desire to improve your marriage
↓
You designate one day in the week for a
"Date night"
↓
You and your spouse feel a deeper and more
committed relationship with one other

- The desire to help your community
↓
You volunteer on weekends to help with the local homeless shelter
↓
You and your family live in a place with a stronger sense of community

- The desire to become the best player on the team
↓
You perform extra reps before and after practice
↓
You help your team win a league championship

Dopamine and Memory

Dopamine has long been understood to have a crucial role in memory, attention, and learning.[4]

The hippocampal–striatal–prefrontal loop that helps orchestrate the formation of new memories relies on dopamine receptors[5].

Scholastic achievement, such as a high grade point average, has been linked to one's dopaminergic system.

---

[4] Yun I, Lee J, Kim SG. Dopaminergic Polymorphisms, Academic Achievement, and Violent Delinquency. Int J Offender Ther Comp Criminol. 2015 Dec;59(13):1409-28. doi: 10.1177/0306624X14554381. Epub 2014 Oct 16. PMID: 25326467.

[5] Clos, M., Bunzeck, N., & Sommer, T. (2019). Dopamine is a double-edged sword: Dopaminergic modulation enhances memory retrieval performance but impairs metacognition. *Neuropsychopharmacology, 44*(3), 555-563. https://doi.org/10.1038/s41386-018-0246-y

Hence the cycle of rewards builds on itself. If one succeeds in school, they may receive academic rewards which could turn into employment opportunities, which could result in financial benefits, and the list goes on.

Deploying Dopamine Effectively

Life is an ongoing journey of growth. The moment you decide to stagnate your personal progress, all sense of purpose becomes lost. It's a commitment you owe to yourself: to constantly aim towards becoming the best version of yourself. Never be satisfied with stagnation and never be satisfied with a wasted day. Each day can be categorized as either a successful one or a wasted one. What separates the two are motivation and dopamine.

A day is all about momentum. People experience a poor night's sleep and instantly forecast a dismal day ahead. Don't let minor defeats derail your ambitions, just as you should never allow modest victories to be overlooked.

Start the morning out strong. Wake up on time. Make your bed. Energize yourself with a cold shower. Confine phone time. Eat a complete breakfast and leave the house on time. Build up that momentum. Build up that dopamine.

You must be willing to make difficult changes in your life. As we said beforehand, it takes a culmination of tweaks to our daily life to begin to see the best versions of ourselves. Attempting weight loss solely through exercise might seem tempting. Spending extensive hours at the gym or braving outdoor runs is a necessary step in weight loss. Yet, this is not the full picture. While expending calories through physical activity is undeniably valuable, it's imperative to recognize that this effort must be complemented by a well-balanced diet and consistency. These factors form the bedrock upon which successful weight loss is built.

Whether it's a small task or a large one, dopamine will urge you to face the next challenge.

Chapter 3
Dopamine's Downfall

Just as we experience spikes in dopamine, we are also susceptible to pronounced drops in its levels.

Every time we have a dramatic spike in dopamine above the baseline, there comes a succeeding drop in dopamine below the baseline.

While addictive behaviors drive their allure by causing increased dopamine levels, a deficiency in dopamine yields considerable impacts on our behaviors as well. If one does not know how to navigate a low dopamine world, they can struggle with their physical and mental health, employment, relationships, and more.

Its ramifications can result in a disruption of many body functions including loss of memory, neurological disorders, and depression. Just as dopamine can play a critical factor in creating motivation, it can just as easily diminish it.

Symptoms of low dopamine include:

- fatigue, stress, and anxiety
- depression
- loss of motivation
- loss of sex drive
- loss of enjoyment in activities that you used to enjoy
- anhedonia (inability to feel pleasure)

Many of these symptoms can lead to other health concerns like obesity, heart disease, struggling relationships, and an overall sense of diminished satisfaction in life.

But even more serious is how dopamine's downfall could lead to our downfall as a species.

Dopamine transcends the idea of being merely a mood enhancer. This single neurochemical has been monumental in the continuation of the human race. Were it not for the motivation that dopamine provided our ancestors- to hunt, protect, and reproduce - we would have not succeeded as a species. Dopamine embodies the much-needed impetus needed to propel humanity forward.

Based On a Reward

When dopamine is released in our brain, its presence changes many neurological aspects of our brain. When you relate a task, especially a difficult one, to a reward earned at the end, you now change the way your brain processes the task. A reward incorporated into any situation becomes a game between intrinsic and extrinsic motivation.

When a reward system is in place, especially through extrinsic motivation, we tend to feel less pleasure while doing that activity. Once we incorporate the prize, our dopamine levels and baseline spike for the reward and not the actual task.

Take a sports team for an example. Each player goes into the season with the hope of winning a championship. Because we automatically relate a reward to mark the end of a challenge, we neurologically change our dopamine systems for the journey ahead. These adaptations induce a delay in the release of dopamine during the pursuit of the reward, in anticipation of its eventual release upon attaining the prize. This reward system creates an overwhelming sensation of fulfillment once overcoming the challenge at the expense of diminished pleasure experienced throughout the journey itself.

The solution to this problem lies within a shift of perspective: transitioning from extrinsic motivation to intrinsic motivation. We'll discuss how to do this in a later chapter.

Advertising

Dopamine is a powerful tool that companies and advertisements use to influence our behavior.

Many of the things we encounter in our daily lives are strategically targeted to stimulate our dopaminergic system. Whether it's food samples at a membership club, the bright sale signs adorning our favorite stores, or the allure of a sizzling cheeseburger on a fast food commercial, these instances exemplify how advertisements tap into our dopamine production.

The art of advertising and manipulation stems from the three E's:
Engage, Educate, and Enlist.

These are used by marketing agencies, healthcare providers, media, and even parents, capitalizing on one's dopaminergic system.

Grabbing the buyer, listener, or audience either by attracting them or *engaging* them allows one to take hold and have them at their attention. Then the seller, radio host, or parent *educates* the captive audience on why their product, advice, or offer is what they need.   Finally, they enlist the person to buy, do as told, or return to listen/view…..and the cycle continues.

For example, When one wants to get their child to eat vegetables they may do the following:

Engage: Do you want to be big and strong like me?
Educate: Well I have muscles because I eat healthy and put vegetables on my plate
Enlist: So eat your vegetables.

In healthcare, we engage in the three E's everyday with patients.. With medical procedures, for example, it may look like this if a
provider needs to convince a patient to have a colon cancer screening by colonoscopy when they declined due to embarrassment

Engage: I had a colonoscopy as well. Wasn't excited about a procedure involving a camera and my colon.
Educate: But there are no other procedures that look at the inside of your colon, have the ability to biopsy a lesion or polyp, and be painless (if sedated) all at the same time such as a

colonoscopy to screen for cancer and diagnose your issues.
Enlist: See the gastroenterologist and discuss the procedure in detail so you can get your concerns addressed.

In advertising, this is also used ubiquitously.

Engage: Red or flashing sale sign to capture the buyer
Educatre: If you come on Saturday you will receive 20% off and save money.
Enlist: So come to the store on Saturday!

These companies conform to a fundamental truth: the more anticipation around a product, the higher the likelihood a customer buys that said product. It's precisely why film studios meticulously edit trailers in a way that showcases the movie's action sequences, iconic actors, and suspenseful lines. These elements capture the audience's attention, drive up the anticipation, and increase the prospect for them to buy a ticket.

This is the same reason why websites buy and sell your data, track your "cookies," and are now using artificial intelligence (AI) for their marketing. The more a business can market to your preferences, the more involved dopamine is with your decision-making process.

Scammers

Millions of Americans are at risk of becoming
victims of fraud. Dating scams, real estate fraud,
and even unnecessary purchases put many of us at
risk for huge financial loss.

Although the average person can spot a scam,
artful criminals know how to prey on us, and they
do it through dopamine.

The trick is very similar to what we see with
gambling. Many find the euphoria of winning or
having a financial gain to be sought after and
replicated.

When many struggle financially and see what they
perceive as a neighbor, friend, or colleague "hitting
it big" on a real estate deal, crypto purchase, or
stock tip, they want to emulate that behavior and
enjoy the same financial gain.

Reports of people believing they are purchasing
real estate that actually doesn't exist, loaning
money to a borrower for high interest who ends up
not existing or paying, or purchasing something
they were manipulated into needing only to find out
they wasted their money pervades society.

Warning Signs of an Investment Scam

Now that you understand how our dopaminergic
system can be manipulated by others, you are in a
much better position to identify the warning signs.
These are some obvious red flags of those who
could be scamming you financially when it comes
to an investment or real estate.

1. Being told to act quickly as "this will be gone
    by tomorrow"
2. Showing pushback when you ask for time to
    research the purchase
3. Inability to locate their valid licenses or
    certifications
4. Being asked to recruit friends or family
    members as potential clients or customers
5. Seeing the term "guaranteed" with a
    concrete percentage. Most investments
    wax and wane over time, so it's unrealistic
    to expect a fixed gain.
6. Language that is confusing and difficult to
    understand
7. Being dissuaded from asking questions or
    being given vague answers.

We all know of someone who got "lucky" with a real
estate buy or business idea and it's perfectly
natural to want to seek that same reward. However
realize, that fraudsters prey upon this and
manipulate our dopaminergic system with verbiage,
numbers, images, and false promises.

Dating/Romance

The first date, the follow-up note, the first kiss, and falling in love ... .all exciting and act like fireworks to our dopaminergic system.

Finding love is one of the biggest dopamine rushes, and people will sometimes do anything to find attention and affection, becoming vulnerable to common dating scams.

Fraudsters may prey upon this, feigning interest, or love, only to later commit financial expenditures from the victim that they never give back.

Hence whether it's diving into an online romance or investment, our advice is to be very careful and do your homework. If it looks and sounds too good to be true, chances are it is too good to be true.

Chapter 4
Dopamine's Role in Addiction

Dopamine plays a pivotal role in shaping our physiological response to addictions. Often perceived as solely a mental health issue, it becomes clear that the addiction cycle including dopamine involves both physiological and biological components. While additions, at first, can become an outlet to relieve pain, continued use will inevitably cause the addiction to become the source of pain.

Much like its ability to make positive actions addicting, dopamine contains a similar influence over negative behaviors as well. Drugs, alcohol, gambling, compulsive eating, and pornography can all activate our dopamine system. Dopamine favors no preference for the specific actions that trigger its release; sometimes causing undesirable habits to become addictive. Essentially, dopamine's quest is to seize the promise of the next reward, and it is willing to embrace risks to attain this goal. Even those who seemingly have the "perfect" life are vulnerable to the destructive nature of addiction, as evidenced by numerous professional athletes squandering their fortunes on gambling and renowned musicians succumbing to substance abuse.

In numerous scenarios, the resurgence of addiction is often triggered by factors revolving around the drug's environment rather than the drug itself. Be it a particular friend or a specific location, the removal of these triggers assumes a pivotal role in the roadmap of rehabilitation, paralleling the significance of other rehab components. Naturally, dopamine emerges as an active player in orchestrating these triggers.

In early incentive salience studies, researchers demonstrated how the urge for a reward is a product of both physiological states and previously ingrained associative behaviors. These studies involved administering a stimulant drug to animals while simultaneously introducing neutral stimuli, such as auditory cues. Initially, dopamine release was tightly tethered to the drug's presence, with no significant response to the neutral stimuli. However, over time, the animals began to react to the sound instead of the drug itself. The animal's neurons ceased their response to the drug's direct influence and instead fired in response to the neutral stimuli associated with it. This means that the animals had a stronger neural reaction to the anticipation of the substance instead of the drug. The mounting anticipation that culminated upon the introduction of the stimulant prompted a surge of dopamine, triggering an intense motivation to seek out the drug.[6]

In essence, dopamine stands as the instigator behind the gradual buildup of anticipation that drives individuals to engage in addictive behaviors.

Let's take porn addiction as another example. Those addicted to pornography dramatically build up their dopamine while engaging in the watching

[6] "THE NEUROBIOLOGY OF SUBSTANCE USE, MISUSE, AND ADDICTION." NCBI, https://www.ncbi.nlm.nih.gov/books/NBK424849/. Accessed 12 August 2023.

of porn. Beyond just visual engagement, their sensory perceptions are also involved, exposing them to an artificial and distorted portrayal of sex. Consequently, individuals grappling with porn addiction may encounter challenges in achieving or sustaining sexual performance during intercourse, a disheartening reality that stems from the dissonance between their dopamine-induced highs during pornography consumption and the muted physical and mental responses during intimate moments.

The ramifications of this predicament extend beyond disappointment in the bedroom. Waning sexual desire can lead to a lack of confidence in social situations, poor motivation to date, and infertility. This preservation serves not only to protect our sexual vibrancy but also to fortify our overall physical well-being, for just as our reproductive capacity is paramount to our existence, so too is ensuring that dopamine dysfunction refrains from negatively changing our holistic health.

Pleasure - Pain Balance

In our daily lives, we are encouraged to pursue pleasure while avoiding pain. Although it seems reasonable to accept this habit, our brains naturally seek to maintain a homeostasis state.

Within this narrative, our body strives to meticulously balance the scales between pleasure and pain. Just as a pleasurable night of drinking is met with a morning hangover, our body finds ways to counterbalance the spectrum of pleasure and pain.

Although we might not realize it, many of us put a lot of emphasis on the pain side where the body wants to regain this balance. Self-imposed pain, such as the example of workaholism, can often masquerade as a constructive addiction, yet its actual implications might be quite the opposite. At times, the weight of excessive labor can unwittingly propel us toward the solace of a drinking binge once the day concludes. Should this become a cycle, the constant shifts between pain and pleasure can lead to extreme stress as our body persistently strives to recalibrate to equilibrium.

Yet, this equilibrium teeters on a delicate edge, particularly when we find ourselves oversaturated by an excess of pleasurable stimuli - making us more susceptible to pain. For instance, taking the phone away from a phone-addicted child would ignite a vicious temper tantrum. Likewise, the tolerance that builds into the life of a drug addict diminishes the potency of the substance while amplifying the feelings of depression and anger during abstinence.

The cognitive dynamics within an addicted mind diverge significantly from those of a typical brain. The hold of addiction can be so unrelenting that abstinence seemingly becomes an insurmountable feat. While onlookers might think, "Why don't they just quit?", the reality is far more complex. Addiction transforms the brain into a perpetual state of dopamine deficiency, where addicts must indulge in their drug not to feel pleasure, but to merely feel normal. These addicts instinctively pursue their drug in the absence of joy and out of complete necessity. Their actions are guided by the urge to restore equilibrium, with the scales perilously tipping towards the side of pain and distress.

With this, the body adopts the universal symptoms of withdrawal which include severe anxiety, depression, and lack of motivation. These symptoms arise as a desperate attempt to realign the internal balance, often pushing the addict back toward the source of their affliction. For them, the return to the addictive substance isn't a matter of seeking pleasure, but instead a matter of mere survival. The natural inclination of our body to restore homeostasis becomes so strong that we willingly go outside of our moral compass to regain a semblance of "normal" sensation.

We have the ability to nurture a harmonious equilibrium between pleasure and pain within our bodies by fostering a well-rounded life. A key aspect of achieving this balance lies in limiting the use of pleasurable stimuli and allowing ample intervals for our body to naturally recover.

It's essential to exercise prudence when the scales tip toward pain. Refraining from pushing our bodies perilously beyond their limits into the realm of danger is crucial. By embracing this mindful stance, we can navigate the intricate balance between pleasure and pain with proper guidance.

Our Addictions

If you have not experienced it yourself, many of us know family members or friends who have struggled with addictions throughout their lives. We see them succumb to their temptations and continually tear themselves down because of it. Painfully, the addictions not only affect the addict but also the family and friends willing to help. When we think of addiction, this is typically the imagery we attribute to it. However, other forms of addiction are a lot harder to recognize. Just because we don't have an ongoing struggle with drugs or alcohol doesn't mean addiction avoids limiting our potential.

Everything in modern life has been made into a drug. Our phones, social media, and apps all create and foster addictive behaviors. A big reason why these substances are so dangerous is because they are accessible to us at all times. Our mornings begin and nights conclude with phone checks, and this device perpetually accompanies our every move. We mindlessly scroll through posts and videos for hours each and every day. These media outlets want you to become addicted. Their platforms are strategically designed to foster addiction, evident in the inevitable request for notification permissions upon app downloads. Each vibration or notification sound triggers a subtle dopamine rush, compelling us to return for further engagement.

Many don't understand that these seemingly unharmful addictions can take the most valuable thing away from us: Time.

Even if an addiction isn't "destroying your life," a strong enough addiction can destroy one's potential in life. Imagine all the time you would have if you continuously make an effort to put your phone down when it is not needed. This time could be used to build better relationships, get extra work done, improve yourself, etc.

Some abuse their dopamine system during addictive activity such that when they recover from their addiction they suffer from severe dopamine imbalance. The system has to thus be "reset" which we will discuss in a later chapter.

Using up all readily available dopamine is also a possibility. This is why those who suffer from addiction seldom achieve much pleasure in any aspect of their life.

Those who suffer from addiction, when indulging themselves in whatever they're dependent on, use up most, and sometimes all, of their available dopamine. This leads to the possibility of no spikes occurring.

This lack of dopamine and inability to rebound can cause one to choose the path of least resistance, going to the action or object from which they receive instant gratification. Hence addictive behavior breeds more addictive behavior without the feeling of "reward".

Chapter 5
Mental Health

Health officials estimate that 1 in 5 adults suffer from a mental health condition.

Being at a dopamine deficit can be a catalyst or result of a mental health issue. Some of the most common mental health conditions affected by our dopamine levels are ADHD, stress, anxiety, and depression.

ADHD

Studies have shown dopamine dysfunction to produce symptoms relating to Attention Deficit/Hyperactivity Disorder (ADHD)[7].

ADHD is a condition in which one may have impulsivity, problems focusing or concentrating, difficulty multitasking, easily distracted, poor organization, issues with prioritizing, becoming frustrated easily, as well as many others.

Criteria for diagnosis of inattention include:

Six or more symptoms of inattention for children up to age 16 years, or five or more for adolescents and adults greater than 17 years old, and symptoms of inattention having been present for at least 6 months, in two more situations (i.e. home, work or school) which include poor listening skills, forgetfulness of daily activities or tasks, poor attention span, being easily distracted or sidetracked, failure to finish or follow through on tasks, avoiding tasks that require significant mental effort, making careless mistakes or inaccuracies, being messy or losing and/or misplacing items needed to complete activities or tasks.[7]

Criteria for diagnosis of hyperactivity include restlessness, squirming when seated or fidgeting with their feet/hands, ability to play or work quietly, and being overly talkative.

Impulsive symptoms include having difficulty waiting for one's turn, frequently interrupting or intruding on others, and impulsivity such as blurting out answers before the questions have been asked.

How dopamine could be a contributor to ADHD symptoms may depend on an increase in dopamine receptors in those with ADHD. Higher dopamine transporter density could result in lower dopamine levels circulating the brain resulting in the above symptoms.[8]

Some studies even show that a considerable amount of ADHD diagnoses are misdiagnosed due to an excess of self-indulgence which causes this drop in baseline dopamine.

[7]Substance Abuse and Mental Health Services Administration. DSM-5 Changes: Implications for Child Serious Emotional Disturbance [Internet]. Rockville (MD): Substance Abuse and Mental Health Services Administration (US); 2016 Jun. Table 7, DSM-IV to DSM-5 Attention-Deficit/Hyperactivity Disorder Comparison. Available from: https://www.ncbi.nlm.nih.gov/books/NBK519712/table/ch3.t3/

[8]Striatal Dopamine Transporter Alterations in ADHD: Pathophysiology or Adaptation to Psychostimulants? A Meta-Analysis Website title: American Journal of Psychiatry

Medical management of ADHD includes stimulants, selective norepinephrine reuptake inhibitors, antidepressants, and alpha-2 adrenergic agonists. Interestingly, many of these medications work by increasing dopamine levels.

Stress and Anxiety

Stress could affect a variety of mental and physical health functions including insomnia, diabetes, anxiety, depression, and even cancer.

When an individual is stressed, they may not know it themselves or convey it to family members directly.

Signs of stress include being quick-tempered, angry, inability to sleep, waking up in the middle of the night, having frequent nightmares, isolating, clinging (in young children), overeating, undereating, making poor choices, memory loss, poor concentration, having a poor attitude towards exercise/sports/school/work, lack of motivation, lack of empathy, headaches, stomach aches, irregular menstruation, weight gain, weight loss, fatigue, hyperactivity, lack of attention to detail, frequent infections, constipation, diarrhea, nausea, vomiting, poor sex drive and erections and more.

Uncontrolled stressors can also induce anxiety.

Social phobia for example has been linked to low dopamine. Those afraid of being around others may become anxious by the unknown that can occur in social settings and will have a hesitancy or phobia of being around others. Social phobia can lead to isolation, poor work performance, poor relationships, and therefore a cycle of low dopamine.

When one has anxiety, they may exhibit insomnia, changes in appetite, mood swings, and at-risk behavior. They may also have an increased heart rate, chest pain, shortness of breath, and more. If one has any of these symptoms they should see a medical provider.

Although some stressors may induce dopamine levels, intense or chronic stressors could inhibit dopamine.

Hence if one wants to improve their dopamine levels, they may need to minimize their stress.

This could be done by eating a well-balanced diet, ensuring adequate sleep, regular exercise, learning to say "No" when it comes to taking on multiple tasks, making small goals rather than setting bars that are unattainable, getting a hobby, being charitable as helping others can be euphoric, talking about what makes you stressed or seek counseling and finding the humor in life, sometimes accomplished by watching short funny movies or videos.

Laughter plays a role in producing and releasing dopamine.[9] Studies have found it to reduce the stress hormone cortisol. In fact, even the anticipation of something being humorous can decrease stress hormones and enhance dopamine's actions.

Hence laughter can be a very effective tool in increasing dopamine.

Schizophrenia

Schizophrenia is a serious mental health condition that has been linked to abnormal levels of dopamine.

Patients with schizophrenia may not only suffer anxiety and depression but also delusions, hallucinations, agitation, repetitive movements, psychosis, and more.

Some of the symptoms incurred in those with schizophrenia are known as "positive" symptoms. These include hallucinations, paranoia, and delusions.

Whereas "negative symptoms" are those in which the patient withdraws, cannot feel pleasure, elicits apathy, and is unmotivated.

---

[9] Anticipating A Laugh Reduces Our Stress Hormones, Study ShowsWebsite title:ScienceDaily

Treatments include therapy, antipsychotics, and medications that may regulate dopamine.

For those exhibiting "positive symptoms", antipsychotic medications that target dopamine are used.

For those exhibiting the "negative symptoms", medications used to stimulate or modulate dopamine are used.

Depression and Suicide

Depression is one of the most common mental health conditions.

Is therefore not surprising that there is a correlation between levels of one's dopamine and depression. Simply, the chance of someone developing depression is higher when dopamine levels are low.

Depression can range from mild to severe. Symptoms include:

- Sadness
- Mood swings
- Irritability
- Lack of motivation
- Insomnia
- Fatigue
- Wanting to avoid others
- Poor appetite

- Diminished interest in activities
- Risk-taking behavior
- Drug use
- Suicidal thoughts and behavior

One of the biggest dangers of dopamine dysfunction is its relationship to suicide.

Studies have found neurobiology could exist in those who contemplate ending their life.

So let's discuss why this could happen.

Each year tens of thousands of Americans take their lives with some reports of an average of 150 people a day. For children and adolescents, suicide is the second leading cause of death.

And each suicide affects everyone with whom the person has regular encounters. So why is it so common? There are multiple reasons why people may choose to end their life.

Firstly, they might not be able to see around the problem. When tragedy strikes, whether it be an accident, break up, job loss, or missed opportunity, some can't see "the light at the end of the tunnel." Many think and navigate through life one step at a time, which may be productive when it comes to tackling tasks, but if they feel the obstacle in front of them is insurmountable they may believe their options are far and few between, with death being the only outcome.

Another reason some consider ending their lives is due to suffering and pain. When one suffers an injury or ages, pain may come in a variety of forms including arthritis, spinal stenosis, cancer metastasis, etc. Yet finding pain control is difficult as medical providers may have long wait times to be seen, face more restrictions in writing opioids, or may not achieve adequate pain control in their patient. Those individuals struggling with pain may tragically look to other options to find relief.

Some suicidal activity might also be linked to impulsive behavior. Many of us have been trained to act on a whim. We quickly reply to a text, pop some food in the microwave, and flick the controller while playing a video game…and these quick, instinctive acts are becoming a part of our daily behavior. So when one has a fleeting thought of suicide, they may be less likely to slow down and think it through.

Another reason some might consider suicide is that they fear death. This is one of the least discussed reasons people commit suicide, but unfortunately more common than we think. Although most of us fear death and dying, some pathologically can't handle the thought of it happening out of the blue. Those who need control and need to plan ahead may find solace in the fact that they are planning their own death.   They can't control their birth but they can control their death, they believe, and for those who feel they have lost control of their life may find this tragic option welcoming.

Loneliness or the feeling of not being cared for can also precipitate suicidal thoughts. Since so many people are undiagnosed when it comes to depression, family members and friends are unaware their loved one is struggling. Going about one's business may be inferred as indifference by someone suffering from a mood disorder. "They won't even notice I'm gone," pervades their thoughts and worsens their loneliness.

Additionally, some consider suicide when they are angry and use it as a form of revenge. If one feels they've been ignored, unheard, or wronged, this could incite an "I'll show 'em" attitude in which their suicide is plotted to be a form of psychological revenge.

Finally, we see suicidal ideation in those who are severely depressed. Some stereotype depression as a person sitting on a couch eating ice cream to combat the tears and loneliness of a breakup. But many have symptoms of severe depression that are less obvious to themselves and family members as mentioned above.

So many self-medicate either by over-eating, drinking alcohol, smoking marijuana, or taking pills. Why? They're trying to increase their "happy hormones" such as dopamine. However, when their alcohol or marijuana wears off, they can sink into a lower funk. Without psychological or medical intervention, one struggles to recover.

Sadly many out there secretly hope they get help but don't know how to ask for it. It's up to us to seek and guide them to a medical professional who can listen, understand, and work with them. Those who are effective at recognizing depression are those who also understand dopamine dysfunction.

Chapter 6
Athletics

When athletes achieve success, we tend to attribute their accomplishments to their training regimens, tireless practice sessions, enduring stamina, and the guidance of skilled coaches. Yet, what often remains obscured from many is the significant role that dopamine takes in bringing athletes success.

A study conducted by researchers at the University of Parma in Italy, featured in the *Journal of Biosciences*, has shed light on the profound influence of dopamine on athletic performance. This investigation delved into the genetic construction of elite athletes' performance. DNA samples obtained from two distinct groups were tested: 50 elite athletes, distinguished by their participation in Olympic or World-level competitions, and 100 control athletes, representing individuals who engage in regular exercise without the competitive context.

The findings unveiled a particularly intriguing insight. Among the four specific genes tested—those associated with muscle development, dopamine transport, cerebral serotonin regulation, and neurotransmitter breakdown—the variance between the two groups was marginal, with one exception. The genes responsible for dopamine transport showcased a notable disparity. The dopamine active transporter exhibited a far higher prevalence and efficiency within the elite athlete cohort compared to their non-competitive counterparts. In fact, the frequency of this transporter was approximately fivefold greater among elite athletes, underscoring its pivotal role in their heightened performance levels.

When it comes to exercise and competition, dopamine plays the following roles:

- Ability to manage pain
- Ability to manage stress
- Ability to endure fatigue and weakness
- Increase motor activity
- Increase endurance
- Motivation
- Increase attention and concentration
- Increase risk-taking

Now you might say, "Wait, risk-taking? Isn't that a part of poor mental health?" We believe in some situations, "risk-taking" is exhibiting the confidence to make it on base, dive toward the end zone, or jump to block a shot in volleyball. Dopamine inspires confidence that allows the athlete to move farther, faster, and put their body on the line when needed. It's the force that imbues athletes with not just the desire to participate in their sport but to transcend boundaries and achieve greatness.

Another role where dopamine plays an effect on athletes is during their retirement or off-season. It's not uncommon to witness retired athletes re-emerge from retirement within a few years, having had a change of heart. Equally, we have also seen ones that end up with severe depression after losing the nature of competition. These circumstances, often referred to as Post-Athletic Activity Depression (PAAD), can manifest when the demanding exercise routines dramatically cease and the psyche isn't adequately prepared to cope with the loss or even being outperformed by fellow athletes. As you will see, biology and psychology play huge factors in the mental health of an athlete.

The unrelenting pressure and inevitable mistakes that sports inherently bring can be a channel for the emergence of depression within athletes. Whether this pressure stems from external forces, such as parental expectations, or arises internally, it fuels an insatiable yearning for success. Additionally, in the aftermath of a challenging match or a taxing season, athletes often intensify the pressure upon themselves to attain the loftier standards they've set for themselves. Many, due to the lowered dopamine levels in the wake of personal setbacks, grapple with heightened self-imposed expectations. Consequently, motivation wanes, rendering the pursuit of excellence a more formidable endeavor.

This process becomes the determining factor that distinguishes average athletes from exceptional ones: the capacity to transform adversity into a catalyst for growth. It's a remarkable ability to convert failure into a learning experience, but one often required to become the best.

Multiple studies have proven that exercise wards off depression. Since we train to be the best, we put our body through physical and mental hardships forcing our dopaminergic systems to work. This is in part due to multiple mood-enhancing hormones being released during athletic activity such as:

- endorphins
- norepinephrine
- dopamine
- serotonin

After a meet, marathon, playoff, or tournament ends, does the average athlete maintain their rigorous training schedule? Probably not. Hence, these hormones that the body has become accustomed to seeing aren't there at their previous levels, inducing depression. If someone is at risk for depression, the drop in these hormone levels could, in theory, depress one to the point that they contemplate suicide.

Being the best puts you psychologically at risk

They say winning is addictive, and this sentiment holds true when viewed through the lens of psychology. Once you win, you reform a new identity. Those who are psychologically mature and grounded don't allow singular victories to define them. Instead, they grasp the fundamental truth that success can only be repeated with continued ambition and work-ethic. Giants like Tom Brady, LeBron James, and Serena Williams would not be etched in history if not for their unwavering pursuit of greatness.

When one ascends to the pedestal of champions, holding that prestigious title, the first-place blue ribbon, or the gleaming gold medal, the world's perception changes—suddenly, you're perceived as "one of the best". How much higher can you go? This crossroad typically offers an athlete two alternatives: to cling steadfastly to their elevated status—a feat made increasingly challenging as one ages and the ascent of ambitious newcomers—or to confront the prospect of decline. What often remains unseen is the exhaustive preparation athletes invest in strategizing for victory. Hours upon hours are dedicated to creating a path to victory, leaving little room for contemplating the prospect of loss. As a result, when the inevitable defeat happens, athletes find themselves unprepared to navigate its emotional aftermath.

What additionally needs to be studied are the mood changes incurred by athletes after each season or race to see if a "funk" sets in because their exercise regimen is not being maintained.

Hence all athletes should have access to counseling to thwart depression caused by losing, being in an off-season, or dealing with the pressure all athletes face at some point in their careers.

Chapter 7
Neurological Disorders

We've established how low dopamine can be devastating to one's mental health. It can also cause severe physical impairment.

Restless Leg Syndrome

Restless Leg Syndrome (RLS) is a condition endured by millions and has been attributed to low dopamine levels[10].

Those with RLS feel leg cramping, pulling, crawling, itching, aching, burning, heaviness, numbness, or a "jumping sensation" in their legs.

They may feel an "overwhelming urge" to move their legs and the uncontrollable sensations and movements can be debilitating.

Although mild cases of RLS occur at night when one is in bed, severe cases could affect a person during the day.

It mimics other neuropathies that cause debilitating leg symptoms.

---

[10] Mitchell UH, Obray JD, Hunsaker E, Garcia BT, Clarke TJ, Hope S, Steffensen SC. Peripheral Dopamine in Restless Legs Syndrome. Front Neurol. 2018 Mar 15;9:155. doi: 10.3389/fneur.2018.00155. PMID: 29599746; PMCID: PMC5862810.

There's been evidence to suggest changes in the basal ganglia could lead to dysfunction in dopaminergic pathways to the peripheral muscles.[11]

Hence treatment includes medications such as ropinirole, pramipexole, and rotigotine to stimulate dopamine.

Parkinson's

Parkinson's disease is the second most common neurodegenerative disorder, next to Alzheimer's, and the most common movement disorder that affects 1% of the world's population over 60 years old. In the US, tens of thousands of new cases are diagnosed each year. It affects several areas of the brain, primarily the substantia nigra, altering balance and movement by affecting dopamine-producing cells.

It was first described in 1817 by James Parkinson as a "shaking palsy."

Common symptoms of Parkinson's include

- Stiffness and rigidity
- Poor balance
- Tremors at rest, especially a pill-rolling tremor
- Slow movement
- Inability to move

[11]Suzuki, K. Microstructural changes in the basal ganglia in restless legs syndrome and migraine. *Sleep Biol. Rhythms* 20, 323–324 (2022). ttps://doi.org/10.1007/s41105-022-00393-6

- Shuffling steps, gait

and patients may later develop…

- Depression
- Anxiety
- Memory loss
- Constipation
- Decreased ability to smell
- Difficulty swallowing
- Erectile dysfunction
- Pneumonia
- Fractures from falling
- Hallucinations
- Delusions
- Dementia

Most cases are idiopathic, meaning the disease arises with no specific cause. However, some cases are genetic, and multiple genes have been identified that are associated with the disease.

The average age of onset is 60, but some cases may occur as "early onset", before the age of 50, and if before the age of 20, it is known as juvenile-onset Parkinson's.

Men appear to be more affected than women at twice the rate.

The risk may be enhanced with a history of head trauma.

Exposure to herbicides and pesticides has been linked to an increased risk of Parkinson's as well.

Although there is no cure for Parkinson's, symptoms can be treated by a variety of measures and many surround improving one's dopamine levels. These include:

- Levodopa – converts to dopamine in the brain, helping replace the deficient hormone.
- Carbidopa (Sinemet) – if given with levodopa prevents the latter from being broken down before it reaches the brain.
- Dopamine agonists – mimic dopamine
- MAO-B inhibitors – help block the enzyme MAO-B, which breaks down natural dopamine
- Other medications including COMT inhibitors, amantadine, and anticholinergics
- Medications to treat anxiety and depression
- Deep brain stimulation – a surgeon implants electrodes into the brain, allowing stimulation of parts that help regulate movement.
- Stem cell therapy – being investigated as a means to create dopamine-producing cells
- Physical and occupational therapy

Pain

Pain is one of the most complex entities of the human body that we've only begun to understand.

Growing evidence has found dopamine to play a role in chronic pain.[12]

Low levels of dopamine have been blamed for the pain those with Parkinson's endure.

With low back pain, for example, studies have found chronic sufferers to have altered dopamine neurotransmission as it relates to pain tolerance and pain sensitivity.

The network of dopamine receptors can play multiple roles in pain modulation as evidenced by those who suffer from chronic pain conditions such as fibromyalgia and neuropathic pain.

Studies have found after an acute episode of pain, dopamine may be released as a defense mechanism to avert behavior that could put one in more harm.

Pain medications such as opioids stimulate dopamine release. This is why opioids are one of the most addictive substances as it easily triggers reward-seeking behavior with their influence on dopamine.

Other drugs that increase dopamine include nicotine, amphetamines, alcohol, and marijuana.

[12] Li C, Liu S, Lu X, Tao F. Role of Descending Dopaminergic Pathways in Pain Modulation. Curr Neuropharmacol. 2019;17(12):1176-1182. doi: 10.2174/1570159X17666190430102531. PMID: 31182003; PMCID: PMC7057207.

These will be later discussed as their addictive nature cannot be overstated.

Interestingly studies have found swearing to help decrease one's pain but were unable to conclude why. It could be a connection between swearing and a surge in dopamine.

Moreover smiling and/or grimacing, such as during a vaccination, has also been linked to tempering the level of pain. Again this could be credited to dopamine.

Modalities that help minimize pain include:
- Applying heat/ice
- Massage
- Physical therapy
- Meditation
- Exercise
- Biofeedback
- Herbs
- Music

and more.

These modalities all have an effect on the dopaminergic system.

Supplements

There are many over-the-counter supplements that can be used to enhance dopamine levels. However, we must understand that the balance between pleasure and pain must also factor into the consideration of substances that directly influence the dopaminergic system. It's notable that nearly every supplement geared toward boosting dopamine production can result in a subsequent crash, alongside a drop in the baseline once the effects of the substance wear off. We therefore urge consulting with one's medical provider before using.

Mucuna Pruriens:

Mucuna pruriens is a tropical bean that grows in parts of Africa, India, and Southern China. This capability stems from its contents of levodopa, a direct precursor to dopamine. Notably, Mucuna Pruriens has exhibited an ability to heighten dopamine production, particularly beneficial for individuals grappling with Parkinson's Disease.

Tyrosine:

Tyrosine, an essential amino acid, is another noteworthy contender in its ability to produce dopamine. Also containing levodopa, Tyrosine plays a pivotal role in facilitating the production of neurotransmitters such as epinephrine, norepinephrine, and dopamine. Typically ingested by pill or powder, Tyrosine has been shown to increase energy levels and enhance focus.

Melatonin:

Interestingly, studies have cast a unique light on melatonin—a hormone frequently associated with sleep regulation. Certain studies have indicated that melatonin might exert a suppressive influence on dopamine production. The utilization of melatonin on a routine basis remains a subject of contention within the scientific community. While the topic is multifaceted, there exists evidence suggesting that melatonin might indeed impact dopamine pathways in an unfavorable way.[13]

[13] Zisapel, Nava. "Melatonin–Dopamine Interactions: From Basic Neurochemistry to a Clinical Setting - Cellular and Molecular Neurobiology." *Springer*, December 2001, https://link.springer.com/article/10.1023/A:1015187601628. Accessed 16 August 2023.

Chapter 8
Obesity

Over 40% of the US population is obese and rising.

With dramatic rises in obesity, scientists have turned to studying the neurological circuits of drug addiction to find how eating habits can activate drug-like behaviors.

Several studies have revealed a significant connection between obesity and a diminished number of dopamine receptors. Consequently, individuals grappling with obesity often seek to augment their dopamine levels by gravitating toward foods that elicit pleasurable sensations.

Some studies have found those with obesity may have fewer receptors for dopamine, hence they try to increase their dopamine by using foods that give them pleasure.

While we know that drug use can spike the body's dopamine levels, addictions can change our dopaminergic system as a whole. Interestingly, this transformative process bears a striking resemblance to obesity, as a high-fat, high-sugar diet will also lead to adaptations in the dopamine system along with the emergence of behaviors similar to addiction.

The act of overconsumption can induce neural plastic changes that exert long-lasting impacts on dopamine signaling. Even after significant weight loss, the altered brain from the prior obesity did not restore normal production. Furthermore, the presence or absence of specific nutrients and their metabolites exerts a direct influence on dopamine release as well.

Multiple studies have also investigated why obesity happens to some and not others.

Factors contributing to obesity include genetics, food choices, high consumption of processed food, poor exercise, and endocrinological disorders such as hypothyroidism.

We've also seen a rise in obesity as more people quit smoking, especially those who had used it to curb smoking.

So, a dopamine deficiency could be spurring poor food choices.

Moreover, as dopamine increases one's motivation, having less of it might affect one's choice to exercise. As stated before, you can put yourself through intense physical workouts, but if you don't continue that motivation to your eating habits, weight loss won't be obtained.

Even though exercise can boost dopamine levels, lack of exercise may cause poor stimulation.

Choosing food to increase dopamine rather than exercise causes a compounding risk for obesity.

Now what about metabolism?

Higher metabolism can cause an increase in calories burned and thus weight loss.

Low metabolism causes a slowing of energy use and can cause weight gain.

Some studies have suggested dopamine affects one's metabolism.

Dopamine not only acts on the central nervous system (brain and spinal cord) and peripheral nervous system but also has been shown to have an influence on the kidneys, immune system, and pancreas.

Focusing on the pancreas, this organ is responsible for multiple functions including the production of insulin to regulate blood sugar.[14]

Studies have found dopamine to increase insulin production. As lower insulin levels lead to high blood glucose and diabetes, dopamine deficiency could be a risk factor for diabetes.

As diabetes is one of the most common illnesses and rising in the pediatric, adolescent, and adult populations, let's break it down.

---

[14] Dopamine Is Key to the Mystery of Metabolic Dysfunction in Psychiatric Patients Website title:Neuroscience News

What is Diabetes?

Diabetes is a disease in which the body doesn't utilize and metabolize sugar properly. When we consume food, it's broken down into smaller components such as proteins, nutrients, fats, water, and sugar. These components are necessary for cell growth and function. They get absorbed in the small intestine and make it to the bloodstream.

In order for a cell to utilize sugar, it needs the hormone insulin to help guide it in. It's similar to a key that fits in the keyhole of the "door" of the cell, opening it up so sugar can enter. Insulin is produced in the pancreas, an organ that receives signals when one eats to release insulin in preparation for the sugar load coming down the pike.

So imagine our mouth like a waiting room, the bloodstream like a hallway, and the cells of the body the rooms along the hallway. Insulin is the key to opening the cells' "doors" allowing sugar to enter. If the sugar does not get in, it stays in the bloodstream "hallway" and doesn't feed the cell. Weight loss occurs, and individuals may become more thirsty as the sugar in the blood makes it fairly osmotic, something the body wants to neutralize, and reduce. The kidneys are going to want to dump the excess sugar, so to do so, one would urinate more, again causing thirst. So when a diabetic loses weight, urinates more frequently, and becomes thirsty, you now understand why.

Complications of Diabetes

Diabetes can cause a multitude of health problems.

These include:

Cardiovascular disease as sugar is sticky, adding to atherosclerotic plaques.

Blindness as high sugar content draws in water to neutralize and small blood vessels in the eye can only take so much fluid before they burst. Moreover, high blood sugar weakens blood vessels.

Kidney disease as the kidneys work overtime to eliminate the excess sugar. Moreover, sugar-laden blood isn't the healthiest when it comes to nourishing our organs.

Infections as pathogens love sugar. It's food for them. Moreover blood laden with sugar doesn't allow immune cells to work in the most opportune environment.

Neuropathy as nerves don't receive adequate blood supply due to the diabetes-damaged blood flow and vessels, hence they become dull or hypersensitive causing diabetics to have numbness or pain.

Dementia as with the heart and other organs, the brain needs healthy blood flow. Diabetes has been found to increase the risk of Alzheimer's as well.

What is insulin resistance?

Insulin resistance, if using our hallway and door analogy, is as if someone is pushing against the door the insulin is trying to unlock. As we know, those with obesity are at higher risk for diabetes, hence fat can increase insulin resistance. It's also been associated with an increase in heart disease.

If your fasting blood sugar (glucose) is greater than 126 mg/dl, or your non fasting blood sugar is greater than 200 mg/dl, you may be considered diabetic. Pre-diabetes occurs when the fasting blood sugar is between 100 and 125 mg/dl. If ignored, and the sugar rises, pre-diabetics may go on to develop diabetes.

However, studies have also found dopamine to cause insulin resistance. Insulin resistance leads to poor blood glucose management and can lead to diabetes.

What also compounds the dopamine/insulin mystery, is studies have found insulin acting on the brain can lower dopamine levels. Hence high circulating insulin could lower one's dopamine, inciting poor food choices, lack of exercise, and thus obesity.

So while science investigates the dopamine/insulin relationship, tips to combat obesity and one's risk of diabetes include:

1. Make exercise not a choice but a daily necessity
2. Eat fresh food and avoid fast food
3. Eat slowly
4. Eat smaller portions.
5. Swap foods high in carbohydrates for vegetables
6. Avoid excessive amounts of sugar in one's diet
7. Monitor your blood sugar

Chapter 9
Learning, Memory, and Sleep

So now you've seen that many of life's challenges could be the result of dopamine dysfunction. Although dopamine dysfunction could lead to severe medical and mental health illness, some of its origins may be subtle, but surmountable.

Learning, memory, and sleep disorders can be signs of dopamine dysfunction and need to be identified and addressed early on.

Memory

It's common for our memory to wane with age, however, individuals of all ages may report changes in their memory.

Memory loss can be attributed to a variety of factors including poor sleep, poor diet, alcohol and drug use, concussions sustained in sports, mental health issues such as depression and anxiety, computer and smartphone use, less hands-on learning, or terminating learning once one graduates from school.

How memory works…

For a memory to be made there must be three processes: encoding, storage, and retrieval.

Encoding works by a multitude of processes that include multiple systems to determine which sense, visual, sound, or experience, for example, will be indexed and stored by the hippocampus, the part of the brain responsible for memory.

Dopamine plays a role in the encoding and consolidation of memories.[15] Moreover, it also plays a role in memory retrieval.

Scientists have described multiple categories of memory including short-term, long-term, sensory memory, working memory, episodic memory, and more.

Dopamine has been found to play a role in multiple memory classifications including short-term, working, episodic, and adaptive.

Likewise, it plays a role as it pertains to memory loss.

Learning

Oftentimes learning is mistaken for "memory". But there is a distinct difference. Learning is the acquisition of a skill or concept that can take time and effort. Creating a memory is a much faster process that allows one to record, store, and then regurgitate information.

---

[15] Clos M, Bunzeck N, Sommer T. Dopamine is a double-edged sword: dopaminergic modulation enhances memory retrieval performance but impairs metacognition. Neuropsychopharmacology. 2019 Feb;44(3):555-563. doi: 10.1038/s41386-018-0246-y. Epub 2018 Oct 25. PMID: 30356095; PMCID: PMC6333779.

Dopamine has been found to play a role not only in memory but the acquisition of learning skills and concepts, hence learning[16].

Dopamine comes into play if the brain finds the act of "learning" to be a reward. To learn, one needs to be motivated to study and put the effort in to acquire the knowledge, hence dopamine is necessary for this to happen.

It can also increase attention span, necessary to focus on what needs to be learned.

Hence those who struggle with attention deficit and learning may find some improvement in dopamine balance.

Smartphone Use

Smartphones and internet use have been linked to memory impairment. Relying on technology to remember phone numbers, perform mathematical calculations, or reach out to family members takes away basic functions our brain performs.

Sleep

Insomnia is a disorder where one has difficulty falling asleep and/or staying asleep. Many factors can cause insomnia including those affected by low dopamine. These may include:

---

[16] The role of dopamine in learning, memory, and performance of a water escape task Website title:Elcenia

- Medications (stimulants, decongestants)
- Caffeine
- Alcohol
- Stress, anxiety, depression
- Thyroid disorder
- Chronic pain
- Neck and back arthritis
- Diabetes
- Respiratory conditions (asthma, COPD)
- Gastroesophageal reflux
- Urinary frequency
- Diarrhea
- Neurological conditions
- Sleep apnea

and of course environmental issues such as noise, temperature, and pets.

Treating insomnia can be complex. We begin by treating the underlying cause, such as any of those listed above. Then we can try the following:

- Lowering the room temperature to an average of 65 degrees F
- Shutting off artificial lights 1-2 hours before going to bed
- Avoiding alcohol
- Eating a dinner including foods rich in tryptophan (fish, nuts, tofu, turkey, eggs and seeds)
- Warm bath
- Cognitive and/or behavioral therapy

- Aromatherapy including lavender
- Blackout curtains to keep out light
- Daily exercise
- Listening to low volume music such as classical or the blues

Now it could be that those who suffer from certain medical conditions are more at risk of insomnia but more needs to be studied in terms of why these medications are linked to poor health outcomes.

Chapter 10
Ways to Improve Dopamine

Enhancing one's dopamine function demands a delicate approach, guided by what we know of this chemical already and proper direction. It is imperative that we navigate this path cautiously, preventing our baseline from escalating to unmanageable heights while pursuing the crucial spikes in dopamine levels that our well-being necessitates. We must pursue sustainable and healthy outlets.

Dopamine, being the impressionable neurotransmitter it is, can be activated by a myriad of triggers. With our understanding of dopamine's intricate effects, it is important that we harness this neuromodulator's potential with utmost efficacy.

Achieving an optimal balance among these variables lies in the act of intermittent dopamine release.

Intermittent Release of Dopamine

The purpose of a proper intermittent release of dopamine is to make ourselves not chase these overwhelming outlets of dopamine rushes.

Randomly Intermittent Reward Timing (RIRT) is an influential schedule that we see constantly. Casinos adroitly use it to sustain the appeal of gambling among addicts, capitalizing on the euphoric feelings associated with winning. Despite many gamblers being aware of the likelihood of losses outweighing victories, the attraction of reliving that pleasure of triumph often overrides rational judgment, prompting prolonged engagement. Similarly, programs use it to keep binge-watchers in front of the television, and video games use it to sustain prolonged gaming sessions. While RIRT is a tool frequently exploited to manipulate our pursuit of pleasure, it can also be harnessed to our advantage.

Even if we aren't gamblers, couch potatoes, or gamers, there is always something in our lives that we do addictively and can be credited to our intermittent dopamine schedule.

Let's take exercise as an example.

The prospect of daily exercise may evoke trepidation in many. To combat this reluctance, we add conditions to our routine—perhaps music, energy drinks, a workout buddy, or the tantalizing promise of a cherished dessert as a reward. We stack many of these dopamine outlets to the point where we don't fear the idea of exercise as much.

However, we've run into times when we forget to bring our earbuds, run out of energy drinks, or our friend cancels out. In such moments, our enthusiasm wanes for the workout, and the driving force that propelled us before becomes absent. This underscores the peril of relying heavily on a multiplicity of factors for creating enjoyment from exercise, where the absence of even one component diminishes that dopamine surge we hope to experience.

To navigate this complex system, it becomes imperative to abstain from over-dependence on a host of dopamine sources. Sustaining an optimal dopamine level for motivation necessitates avoiding consistent, unsustainable spikes while embracing the inherent variability of the spikes we encounter. This strategic approach ensures that our dopamine baseline remains within manageable levels, delivering a sustained state of gratification and pleasure.

By consciously curbing your phone usage during social interactions or forsaking music during your morning walks, you can proficiently modulate your dopamine usage. This strategic trimming of dopamine enhancers potentially results in a heightened appreciation for these experiences over the long haul.

Interestingly, caffeine is one of the few stimulants that is the exception to this rule.

Caffeine ingestion upregulates dopamine receptors and makes the body more sensitive to dopamine's effect even if levels are low.

However, this applies only to unadulterated caffeine, not energy drinks. Energy drinks contain many other influencers, such as taurine, that can uncontrollably cause dopamine levels to spike. The recommended threshold for caffeine intake in healthy individuals ranges from 100 to 400 mg a day. Levels above 400 mg are not recommended and could be linked to adverse effects.

Inevitably, the sustained elevation of dopamine levels during specific activities—be it work, exercise, or personal pursuits—can also degrade motivation for those very tasks over time. This phenomenon, although gradual, eventually produces a decline in both pleasure and motivation associated with these endeavors.

So, the question remains: How can we prudently heighten our dopamine levels? The answer lies within cultivating sound health habits, encompassing exercise, diet, and proper supplementation.

Extrinsic to Intrinsic Motivation

As discussed in Chapter 2, when we integrate a task with a physical reward, we lose pleasure in the journey. Solely focusing on that semester grade, championship trophy, or end-of-the-year bonus will undermine the dopamine process for the task. To resolve this, we must change our extrinsic motivation to intrinsic motivation.

One approach to achieve this transformation is through a subtle self-deception. We change our thinking to wherein we persuasively convince ourselves that we derive gratification from the toil and exertion, independent of any external reward. Many social media influencers praise this way of thinking. (Though, it's important to note that achieving an intrinsic embrace of discomfort, as portrayed by these influencers, might often be an ambitious aspiration beyond immediate reach.)

Through this mental adjustment, we possess the ability to reprogram our neural circuitry, inducing the release of dopamine exclusively during the exertion phase, rather than prematurely or post-event. This intentional rewiring serves to regulate the dopamine spikes while forestalling an unwarranted escalation of our threshold.

Cold Exposure

Cold exposure has emerged as a contemporary trend within the realm of fitness, urging enthusiasts to relinquish their cherished warm showers in favor of invigorating cold water immersions and ice baths. This phenomenon has been propelled into the public eye by influential media figures, championing the benefits of subjecting oneself to cold temperatures. This exposure to cold temperatures has been found to increase dopamine production and norepinephrine. In fact, these ice baths used by athletes have been found to increase dopamine levels by 250%.[17] The dopamine increase one experiences during an ice bath can be the same magnitude as the experience of doing cocaine. However, the distinction lies in the distinctive trajectory of dopamine's release—whereas drug-induced highs entail an abrupt ascent and crash, cold therapy instigates a gradual, sustained rise in dopamine levels over subsequent hours. This dopamine release often translates into a prolonged uplift in mood, persisting

---

[17] Srámek P, Simecková M, Janský L, Savlíková J, Vybíral S. Human physiological responses to immersion into water of different temperatures. Eur J Appl Physiol. 2000 Mar;81(5):436-42. doi: 10.1007/s004210050065. PMID: 10751106.

well beyond the conclusion of the cold exposure exercise.

It's imperative to exercise caution when approaching cold therapy, as exposure to low temperatures carries inherent risks such as body heat loss, hypothermia, frostbite, shock, and in severe cases, even fatality. Hypothermia, marked by a perilous drop in body temperature, can manifest swiftly, with signs emerging at temperatures of 95 degrees Fahrenheit—triggering shivering, accelerated respiratory and heart rates, and cognitive confusion.

Another consideration for one's morning routine should be sun exposure. Not only has sunlight been linked to better quality sleep at night, but has also shown a positive correlation to dopamine. Exposure to sunlight within the first hour of the day can cause a maintained level of dopamine similar to taking a cold shower.

One should consult a healthcare professional on how to balance healthy sunlight exposure and skin cancer risk.

Exercise

Dopamine levels can be increased with as little as 10 minutes of aerobic exercise.[18] Regular exercise and slowly increasing intensity or length of workouts can have some beneficial effects.

---

[18] Hansen CJ, Stevens LC, Coast JR. Exercise duration and mood state: how much is enough to feel better? Health Psychol. 2001 Jul;20(4):267-75. doi: 10.1037//0278-6133.20.4.267. PMID: 11515738.

Most medical groups suggest at least 150 minutes of moderate to vigorous exercise each week to protect one's health and lower the risk of chronic disease.[19]

Exercise intensity and duration should also be verified with one's healthcare provider.

Diet

Our diet plays a crucial role in boosting dopamine levels.

Phenylalanine and tyrosine comprise two initial steps in the biosynthesis of dopamine. Hence as dopamine is made from these two precursors, those foods rich in tyrosine and phenylalanine can increase one's dopamine levels.

Foods that therefore increase dopamine include:

- Green leafy vegetables
- Chicken
- Beef
- Turkey
- Fish (such as salmon and mackerel)
- Green tea
- Dark chocolate
- Beets
- Avocados
- Apples

---

[19] Physical Activity Guidelines for Americans, 2nd edition Website title:Office of Disease Prevention and Health Promotion

- Bananas
- Eggs
- Nuts (such as almonds, walnuts)
- Sesame and pumpkin seeds

As you see many of these foods are rich in vitamins and healthy, well-balanced diets have been found to improve not only physical health but mental health including dopamine levels.

Not only can foods play a role but supplements have been studied on their ability to enhance dopamine levels.

These include:

- Niacin (B3)
- Vitamins B5 B6
- Folate (B9)
- Vitamin D
- Magnesium
- Gingko
- L-theanine
- Ginseng
- Omega-3 essential fatty acids
- Probiotics
- Turmeric
- Iron

Senses, Music, and Meditation

Research has also investigated how our senses can stimulate dopamine receptors.[20]

Hence not only could the above foods and supplements stimulate dopamine release but actual taste bud stimulation, such as sweet or sour flavors.

Certain smells can increase dopamine. These include lavender, citrus such as lemon, and bergamot.

Vision is another sense that can increase dopamine. For example, visual stimuli that evoke a good memory and or happy thoughts can stimulate dopamine.[21] Moreover, studies have found light stimuli, such as flickering lights, to affect dopamine release. This includes light exposure later in the day and before sleep. It's recommended to dim or completely turn off bright lights in the home a few hours prior to going to sleep.

Sounds of course can help induce dopamine levels such as music and even non-melodic frequencies.

And finally, the sense of touch is not without its dopamine-inducing role. Touch such as hugging and holding has been found to tell the brain to release oxytocin which can in turn stimulate dopamine.

---

[20] Katz DB, Sadacca BF. Taste. In: Gottfried JA, editor. Neurobiology of Sensation and Reward. Boca Raton (FL): CRC Press/Taylor & Francis; 2011. Chapter 6. Available from: https://www.ncbi.nlm.nih.gov/books/NBK92789/

[21] Eleanor Dommett et al. ,How Visual Stimuli Activate Dopaminergic Neurons at Short Latency.Science307,1 476-1479(2005).DOI:10.1126/science.1107026

Yoga can be practiced to help improve dopamine
levels. Some studies have found one hour of yoga
daily for three months to significantly increase
dopamine levels.[22]

Meditation not only provides multiple benefits
including relaxation but studies have shown it to
increase dopamine as well.

Massage is another modality that has positive
effects on dopamine while improving relaxation and
stress relief.

Staying active and limiting computer/smartphone
use is a given. As screen time has been found to
cause surges of dopamine but then desensitize our
brain to it, limiting indoor activities with screens and
being more active can improve dopamine. Studies
have shown that screen time and bright lights
before bed not only disrupt sleep patterns but also
have a long-lasting effect on dopamine levels.

Pets can become our best friends the moment they
get adopted, or adopt us. Studies have shown
petting a dog or having a pet increases dopamine.
Whether it's the love, touch, or the need to walk
them and stay active, pets can be a huge help
when it comes to dopamine levels. Actively
engaging with someone you have a strong
relationship with has also been linked to dopamine
surges.

[22] Pal R, Singh SN, Chatterjee A, Saha M. Age-related changes in cardiovascular system, autonomic functions, and levels of BDNF of healthy active males: role of yogic practice. Age (Dordr). 2014;36(4):9683. doi: 10.1007/s11357-014-9683-7. Epub 2014 Jul 11. PMID: 25012275; PMCID: PMC4150910.

Laughter is one of nature's antidotes to sadness and "infusion" of good feelings. Laughter not only helps release dopamine but swaps it for the stress hormone cortisol. Finding humor in life seems difficult when one is fatigued, depressed, or stressed, but fortunately, there are troves of content within movies, TV shows, videos, memes, social media, and one's friends that can make one smile, giggle, and laugh.

Music has long been studied as it pertains to its effect on mood and has been strongly linked to dopamine surges.[23] And it doesn't necessarily have to be a song one likes. Multiple types of sounds and tones can stimulate the neurotransmitter and if one plays an instrument or dances to the music, the dopamine benefit surges more.

---

[23] Ferreri L, Mas-Herrero E, Zatorre RJ, Ripollés P, Gomez-Andres A, Alicart H, Olivé G, Marco-Pallarés J, Antonijoan RM, Valle M, Riba J, Rodriguez-Fornells A. Dopamine modulates the reward experiences elicited by music. Proc Natl Acad Sci U S A. 2019 Feb 26;116(9):3793-3798. doi: 10.1073/pnas.1811878116. Epub 2019 Jan 22. PMID: 30670642; PMCID: PMC6397525.

Chapter 11
Deploying Dopamine

Triumph emerges for those unafraid to tread the challenging path.

This difficulty we endure, although viewed by some as unnecessary, is what many of us hope to not only conquer but to continually pursue.

In the contemporary world, an overwhelming emphasis seems to rest on traversing the course of least resistance. Worryingly, the number of individuals intentionally subjecting themselves to more arduous circumstances than life necessitates is dwindling. Today's landscape diverges remarkably from any other era. With a wealth of resources and knowledge at our disposal, modern humans possess the capability to shape any quality of life they wish. The trajectory towards a fulfilling existence is open to anyone willing to navigate it. The hardship lies in assimilating the discipline to embrace obstacles, opting to delay instant gratification in favor of a more profound, future-forged fulfillment. Developing a life suffused with seemingly inconsequential habits, which may appear shallow initially, forms the cornerstone of building an empire in time to come.

A sad reality in the modern world is the tendency to regard those striving for robust physical and mental well-being as extremists. We scoff at people who voluntarily wake up before the sun rises or continue to work well late into the night. These individuals are driven by an unmatched desire for health, success, and a prolonged, vibrant life. While it's true that some might push their physical boundaries to a dangerous extent, the message here isn't to adopt every challenge they undertake. Instead, it's an invitation to adopt wisdom from their mindset rather than categorize them as outsiders.

Rather than recoiling from life's hardships, they should be embraced as opportunities for personal growth. It's an opportunity to acquaint oneself with the experience of physical and mental discomfort, and subsequently, master the art of overcoming it.

This endeavor demands a steadfast, unwavering motivation. It is through the work of dopamine that the seemingly unattainable can indeed be achieved.

Through the adoption of these changes, the improvements we desire become discernible. Be it financial, physical, social, or psychological pursuits, dopamine becomes our greatest asset in propelling us toward our aspirations.

References

1. Oleson, Erik B., and Joseph F. Cheer. "A Brain on Cannabinoids: The Role of Dopamine Release in Reward Seeking." *National Library of Medicine*, 2012. https://www.ncbi.nlm.nih.gov/pmc/articles/PMC3405830/. Accessed 27 July 2023.

2. Buchholz, Katharina. "Chart: America's Top New Year's Resolutions for 2023." Statista, 23 December 2022, https://www.statista.com/chart/29019/mos t-common-new-y ears-resolutions-us/. Accessed 7 August 2023.

3. Batts, Richard. "Why Most New Year's Resolutions Fail | Lead Read Today | Lead Read Today." Fisher College of Business, 2 February 2023, https://fisher.osu.edu/blogs/ leadreadtoday/why-most-new-years-resoluti ons-fail. Accessed 7 August 2023.

4. Yun I, Lee J, Kim SG. Dopaminergic Polymorphisms, Academic Achievement, and Violent Delinquency. Int J Offender Ther Comp Criminol. 2015 Dec;59(13):1409-28. doi: 10.1177/0306624X14554381. Epub 2014 Oct 16. PMID: 25326467.

5. Clos, M., Bunzeck, N., & Sommer, T. (2019). Dopamine is a double-edged sword: Dopaminergic modulation enhances memory retrieval performance but impairs metacognition. Neuropsychopharmacology, 44(3), 555-563. https://doi.org/10.1038/s41386-018-0246-y

6. "THE NEUROBIOLOGY OF SUBSTANCE USE, MISUSE, AND ADDICTION." NCBI,

https://www.ncbi.nlm.nih.gov/books/NBK42 4849/. Accessed 12 August 2023.

7. Volkow ND, Wang G, Kollins SH, et al. Evaluating Dopamine Reward Pathway in ADHD: Clinical Implications. JAMA. 2009;302(10):1084–1091. doi:10.1001/jama.2009.1308

8. Substance Abuse and Mental Health Services Administration. DSM-5 Changes: Implications for Child Serious Emotional Disturbance [Internet]. Rockville (MD): Substance Abuse and Mental Health Services Administration (US); 2016 Jun. Table 7, DSM-IV to DSM-5 Attention-Deficit/Hyperactivity Disorder Comparison. Available from: https://www.ncbi.nlm.nih.gov/books/NBK51 9712/table/ch3.t3/

9. Striatal Dopamine Transporter Alterations in ADHD: Pathophysiology or Adaptation to Psychostimulants? A Meta-Analysis Website title:American Journal of Psychiatry

10. Anticipating A Laugh Reduces Our Stress Hormones, Study Shows Website title:ScienceDaily

11. Filonzi L, Franchini N, Vaghi M, Chiesa S, Marzano FN. The potential role of myostatin and neurotransmission genes in elite sport performances. J Biosci. 2015 Sep;40(3):531-7. doi: 10.1007/s12038-015-9542-4. PMID: 26333399.

12. Mitchell UH, Obray JD, Hunsaker E, Garcia BT, Clarke TJ, Hope S, Steffensen SC. Peripheral Dopamine in Restless Legs Syndrome. Front Neurol. 2018 Mar 15;9:155.

doi: 10.3389/fneur.2018.00155. PMID: 29599746; PMCID: PMC5862810.

13. Suzuki, K. Microstructural changes in the basal ganglia in restless legs syndrome and migraine. Sleep Biol. Rhythms 20, 323–324 (2022). ttps://doi.org/10.1007/s41105-022-00393-6

14. Li C, Liu S, Lu X, Tao F. Role of Descending Dopaminergic Pathways in Pain Modulation. Curr Neuropharmacol. 2019;17(12):1176-1182. doi: 10.2174/1570159X17666190430102531. PMID: 31182003; PMCID: PMC7057207.

15. Zisapel, Nava. "Melatonin–Dopamine Interactions: From Basic Neurochemistry to a Clinical Setting - Cellular and Molecular Neurobiology." Springer, December 2001, https://link.springer.com/article/10.1023/A:1015187601628. Accessed 16 August 2023.

16. Scientists Find Link Between Dopamine And Obesity Website title:ScienceDaily

17. Dopamine and glucose, obesity, and reward deficiency syndrome Website title:Frontiers

18. Dopamine Is Key to the Mystery of Metabolic Dysfunction in Psychiatric Patients Website title:Neuroscience News

19. Clos M, Bunzeck N, Sommer T. Dopamine is a double-edged sword: dopaminergic modulation enhances memory retrieval performance but impairs metacognition. Neuropsychopharmacology. 2019 Feb;44(3):555-563. doi: 10.1038/s41386-018-0246-y. Epub 2018 Oct 25. PMID: 30356095; PMCID: PMC6333779.

20. The role of dopamine in learning, memory, and performance of a water escape task Website title:Elcenia

21. Srámek P, Simecková M, Janský L, Savlíková J, Vybíral S. Human physiological responses to immersion into water of different temperatures. Eur J Appl Physiol. 2000 Mar;81(5):436-42. doi: 10.1007/s004210050065. PMID: 10751106.

22. Hansen CJ, Stevens LC, Coast JR. Exercise duration and mood state: how much is enough to feel better? Health Psychol. 2001 Jul;20(4):267-75. doi: 10.1037//0278-6133.20.4.267. PMID: 11515738.

23. Physical Activity Guidelines for Americans, 2nd edition Website title:Office of Disease Prevention and Health Promotion

24. Katz DB, Sadacca BF. Taste. In: Gottfried JA, editor. Neurobiology of Sensation and Reward. Boca Raton (FL): CRC Press/Taylor & Francis; 2011. Chapter 6. Available from: https://www.ncbi.nlm.nih.gov/books/NBK92789/

25. Eleanor Dommett et al. ,How Visual Stimuli Activate Dopaminergic Neurons at Short Latency.Science307,1476-1479(2005).DOI:10.1126/science.1107026

26. Pal R, Singh SN, Chatterjee A, Saha M. Age-related changes in cardiovascular system, autonomic functions, and levels of BDNF of healthy active males: role of yogic practice. Age (Dordr). 2014;36(4):9683. doi: 10.1007/s11357-014-9683-7. Epub 2014 Jul 11. PMID: 25012275; PMCID: PMC4150910.

27. Ferreri L, Mas-Herrero E, Zatorre RJ, Ripollés P, Gomez-Andres A, Alicart H, Olivé G, Marco-Pallarés J, Antonijoan RM, Valle M, Riba J, Rodriguez-Fornells A. Dopamine modulates the reward experiences elicited by music. Proc Natl Acad Sci U S A. 2019 Feb 26;116(9):3793-3798. doi: 10.1073/pnas.1811878116. Epub 2019 Jan 22. PMID: 30670642; PMCID: PMC6397525.

28. Huberman, Andrew. "Controlling Your Dopamine For Motivation, Focus & Satisfaction | Huberman Lab Podcast #39." YouTube, 27 September 2021, https://www.youtube.com/watch?v=QmOF0 crdyRU&ab_channel=AndrewHuberman.